Walking for Fitness

A Comprehensive Guide on How Walking can improve your Health and Well-being Forever

By
Faye Froome

Faye Froome **Copyright © 2016**

Table of Contents

Introduction

Exercise doesn't have to be difficult. Anything that raises the heartbeat above a resting state can be considered exercise including an activity that most of us overlook – walking. Walking is the perfect solution to most of our weight and fitness struggles, as it is free, easy, satisfying and suitable for all ages and weight groups.

This guide will provide you will a thorough introduction into everything you need to know about walking for fitness, such as how to avoid, recognize and deal with common injuries, how to stay hydrated, prepare for long distance walking and much, much more.

I bet many of you have taken a few hundred or even a thousand or more steps already today, see we told you it was easy, you're exercising without even realizing it.

All many of us need to do to turn a few more steps into an effective exercise regime is make a few small changes to our daily routine. In fact these changes are so small that many of us could do them with even thinking about it. It really is that easy.

So forget about buying that expensive exercise equipment, signing up to monthly gym membership fees, and trying the latest fad diet and get your walking shoes on instead and walk your way to a fitter and healthier you.

By the end of this guide you should be prepared to take up a new walking regime. So what are you waiting for let's get going, let's get fit, and most importantly lets have fun!

Chapter 1 – Walking Basics

Benefits of Walking

It's common for people who want to become fitter to start going to the gym or join a sport club. Yet there is an easier and gentler way to improve your fitness, a method which you use everyday – walking.

Nearly all of us are fortunate enough to be able to walk, and as a hobby it has almost no other requirements. There are no monthly membership costs, no physical or emotional commitments and little to no equipment you really need above a good pair of shoes.

Walking, although not always considered a form of exercise, still retains most of the benefits from a good workout. You can burn away a considerable amount of calories and work towards a healthier weight.

You can kick start your metabolism, which will also improve your energy levels, help bolster your immune system and mitigate various diseases and illnesses that can occur due to poor diet (such as diabetes). Walking also contributes to our overall mental health, helping you unwind after a long day, improving your sleep patterns and contributing to self-esteem and confidence.

Furthermore walking is also easy to incorporate into our life. Most of us can, at some point of the day, include a gentle walk, whether this is during a lunch break, in the evening or used as a form of transport.

Walking carries a lower risk of injury than almost every other form of exercise making it a fantastic form of exercise for older adults. As humans we are physically designed to walk and run.

How often should I walk?

National guidelines suggest that you need at least 150 minutes of moderate intensity exercise every week to stay healthy. This is a good benchmark to work towards; however as exercise is defined as moderate intensity, it should only include *brisk* walking. Of course longer duration walking will improve your fitness and health, although there are no national guidelines detailing the benefits of lower intensity but longer duration exercise vs. higher intensity short exercise.

With that being established, there is no need to limit yourself to just 150 minutes – you can walk as far as you like. One of the many benefits of walking compared to other forms of exercise is the ease of performing longer walking sessions with less strain, injury, and effort.

Calories Used
So you may be wondering - how many calories does walking actually expend? How does it compare to other forms of exercise?

In response to the first question, it correlates with the weight of the person walking. People who are heavier will burn more calories as they walk, because they require more energy to move. Similarly, the level of incline can also affect calorie expenditure, which sharper inclines requiring more energy to traverse. Even factors such as the quality of your shoes and your walking technique can be influential in your ability to burn energy.

Walking at a faster rate also burns more energy than walking slower, due to the various additional metabolic processes that occur at more intense levels of activity. Sweating, increasing breathing rate and circulation all force the body to expend more energy than just the energy required than the energy used moving.

Owing to this, a precise figure is hard to determine, although many websites across the internet can provide various estimates. Let's for example use the website, mapmywalk.com to estimate the calorie expenditure for a *brisk* walk. The average speed of walking for most humans is between 3-4 miles per hour, so let's presume a brisk walker may be able to cover up to 6 miles in an hour, or roughly 10 minutes per mile.

According to mapmywalk.com, for a 175 lb, 5ft 8, 30 year old male a 1 mile walk in 10 minutes will burn approximately 145 calories.

Alternatively, for 135 lb 5ft. 6, 30 year old female who walks 1 mile in 10 minutes, 114 calories are burned.

To put this in perspective the recommended calorie intake for men and women is 2500 and 2000 calories respectively. A mere 30 minutes of brisk walking gives us an approximate calorie expenditure of 435 and 342 calories for us theoretical average man and theoretical average women. That's 17.4% and 17.1% of your total energy intake burned – not bad for a mere 30 minutes of walking.

Furthermore, as previously mentioned, these values will increase the heavier you are, increasing the potential of walking as a weight loss solution.

It is thought that a pound of body fat is roughly equal to around 3500 calories. Several scientists have argued this figure is mildly inaccurate; however it can be useful as an estimate to consider. Using our previous estimates of 342-435 calories for our average brisk walker, this gives us a very rough and crude estimate of losing about 1 lb every 8-10 days. It is not a staggering level of weight loss, but nor is it insignificant. Furthermore it is likely to be far more sustainable than fad diets and brutal eating regimes most of us endorse when we are trying to lose weight.

Walking Compared To Running

For many people the question isn't whether they should walk or not, it is whether they should be walking or running. Both forms of exercise have many benefits, but ultimately, this doesn't make them equal. Running does burn notably more calories than walking, with some sources approximately 2.5 times more calories burned during a run compared to walk over the same distance.

There is also evidence to suggest that running is better in terms of the neuro-chemical and hormonal changes it produces on the body. For example some studies have reported that running leads to more weight loss than walking, even when the calorie expenditure for both forms of exercise was equivalent. Likewise some studies have also suggested that running improves appetite management and has a greater impact on depression.

Of course, running is harder both physically and mentally and for many people, to start with walking is a necessity, not a choice. Running also has a dramatically higher chance of injury, even for people with a good technique. Walking still has well-documented and established benefits for weight, blood sugar and diabetes.

Overall, if you are desperate to burn calories on a timeframe, running might be a better choice. Likewise if you want to transform your body rapidly, running has its advantages. Nonetheless, walking is often more practical and easier to maintain, typically leading to greater consistency of exercise over time for the casual exerciser.

As we all have to walk rather than run you can see the obvious advantage in maintaining a walking regime, we all do it already!

Walking & Safety

Although walking is a gentle activity, it is still wise to adhere to safety precautions as you walk. You should always take a drink with you when you walk, especially for longer walks and during hotter days. This drink will preferably be cold water, but any refreshing fluid will do, but try and avoid sugary sports branded drinks.

It is also a good idea to inform people that you are out for a walk. This ensures that someone will pay attention if you do not come back, perhaps due to getting lost or being injured. This is particularly important if you favor walking in rural trails where you might not encounter other people and the path may be cobbled or difficult to walk on.

It can also be considered important during late night walks where it is easier to become lost or encounter trouble. If possible it can be good idea to walk with at least one other person or in a group.

Consider the neighborhood. Stick to areas that are known to be safe and have plenty of activity during the hours you chose to walk. Avoid dangerous areas where there a few people about. Likewise, avoid wearing or displaying unnecessary valuables, such as expensive jewelry whilst walking which can draw undesired attention.

It is always best to know your route in advance. If you chose a walking route which you are not familiar with, ensure you bring with you a map or mobile GPS to help you in case you lose your way.

Although many people enjoy listening to music during their walk it is often better to avoid music as it distracts you from your surroundings, meaning you are delayed in your reactions to dangerous situations. If you must listen to music as you walk, use a low volume setting or only use a single earphone.

Likewise it is also a good idea to always keep a mobile phone on your person as well as a small amount of money to get yourself out of any difficulties you might face. Enough for a taxi fare should suffice.

Wearing brighter clothing is also advised. This allows you to be easily seen by oncoming vehicles and other pedestrians. During the evening, reflective clothing is particularly important as normal brighter colors might not be easily identified.

If you must walk on a road without any pavement, always ensure you are walking into oncoming traffic, rather than away from it. This ensures that you can always see what vehicles that are coming towards you and allows you to avoid any vehicles that are not driving safely. If your back is facing oncoming traffic there is a significant risk a wayward driver may hit you in the rear.

How to Start

Start gradually. Begin by taking a slow and short walk of around 10-15 minutes. Of course, most people will be able to walk significantly faster and for significantly longer than 15 minutes, but starting small has numerous advantages. By starting small, you allow yourself to form a habit through consistent practice. It is more important to consistently do a small walk than perform larger walks with irregularity. Generally speaking, the former will also amount to a greater distance, which is crucial if you are using walking as a means for weight loss.

At only 15 minutes a day you should easily be able to walk every day, with no excuse as to why you cannot fit walking into your schedule. At this stage it's not important to dwell on your technique or your distance, just getting into the habit is the most important thing. After all, 15 minutes a day amounts to 1hr & 45 minutes per week – a sizeable amount of exercise.

After a few weeks, you can start to develop your walking practice further. Walking slowly will also allow you to focus on factors such as pace and posture. The correct posture assumes an elongated, but not entirely rigid spine. You should walk with an upright rigidness – if your back is forced to be straight, your back muscles will feel the strain rather quickly.
Good posture, when practiced, should be effortless. Let's face it we have been walking since we were toddlers so a good walking posture should already be defined, or requires minimal adjustment.

Also focus on pace. You want to walk with a regular speed. This helps you regulate your intensity, choosing a pace that you can maintain, but at the same time presents a little challenge when held for a longer period of time. It also helps you consider your timing and your distance – if you walk at a regular pace you will be able to intuitively know how far you have walked and how fast.

In terms of fitness, a good pace starts as what is commonly termed a 'talking pace'. At this pace your breathing is elevated, but you would still be able to hold a conversation and talk with someone else whilst walking alongside them.

Once you have both good posture and pace established, you can then increase the duration of time you are walking for. Thirty minutes per day will have an impact on your general fitness, at least if you establish a talking pace.

If you are looking for higher levels of fitness and keeping your walk at around 30 minutes you should be looking at increasing the pace so that your breathing becomes hard, although not strained.

For weight loss, longer periods of walking are recommended. 60 minutes a day at a talking pace will cause a significant amount of calories to be burned.

The Importance of Variety

Don't presume that your walks need to be in rural areas or designated walking paths – there are so many interesting and unique routes that can be undertaken in urban areas. Do a little research and look up your local area – often you will be surprised at just how much is available to walk around. Often it is quite embarrassing – we can live in a place for several years without realizing the wealth of routes and interesting features in the surrounding regions.

Most of us will also probably live within walking distance from our jobs. However we won't necessarily think its walking distance but if its 3km or less it's definitely a great option to increase your walking activity. Incorporating walking in to your daily routine can pay massive dividends towards reaching ones goals.

Also embrace opportunities that give you more potential to walk. Volunteering, especially in a natural setting, joining walking or rambling groups or walking with your kids in parks are also easy and relaxed ways you can increase your walking count.

Establish Goals

A common goal is to walk around 10,000 steps per day. This goal doesn't have to be your specific goal, however, it is useful to establish other goals during your practice, which will help keep you motivated and disciplined.

For example, walking around 1,000 steps in 10 minutes is a reasonable standard of walking for a regular person. Consider timing your walks to try and accomplish walking at this pace.

Also consider staggering your walking periods throughout the day. Accomplishing a few thousands steps in the morning, a few thousand more during the day and finally a few thousand more in the evening is typically easier than doing 10,000 in one setting.

Mall Walking

In order to help increase public fitness, mall walking is increasingly encouraged across the U.S.

Mall walking alleviates many of the concerns and difficulties associated with outside walking whilst still retaining the benefits. Malls typically are temperature controlled, ensuring that they are neither too hot nor too cold. Malls also have protection from the elements, helping you to avoid intense sunlight, rain and wind.

Furthermore malls have security staff and plenty of other people present in the area. This can ensure you feel safe and secure during your walking exercise. Malls are also often easy to walk in, as you are unlikely to slip, trip or fall on the flat and textured mall surfaces compared to rocky and uneven natural settings.

Malls also have a few special conveniences. They have restrooms and places to buy snacks and refreshments. They even have shops to sell fitness gear just in case you need to pick up a replacement pair of walking shoes or a new backpack.

Owing to this, mall walking and mall walking programs can be a fantastic choice for people who do not enjoy walking outdoors but can't afford or do not feel comfortable in a gym setting.

Chapter 2 – Hydration & Nutrition

Water & Walking

It's always important to take enough fluids with you when you walk, but how much is enough? Is a simple water bottle enough or do you need an entire flagon?

The answer depends on how intense your walking is. We drink water to replace fluids that we lose during the day. Some of this fluid is lost as urine, some of it is through the skin drying out but some is also lost through sweating.

Sweating helps us control our temperature, keeping us in the biological sweet spot of 37-38 degrees. If our body temperature rises too high your cells start to become stressed and even die, so regulating body temperature is essential to our survival. When you become dehydrated during exercise you lose this ability to regulate your temperature and risk heat exhaustion.

During an intense walk, especially during a hot day, you will sweat a lot to control your temperature. In fact, during the most intense periods of exercise the amount you sweat will rapidly exceed the amount of water your body can biologically absorb.

Isotonic drinks can be helpful to mitigate risk of dehydration. Isotonic drinks contain special substances that help our body increase the uptake of fluids. They also tend to contain small amounts of sugar to help maintain performance during exercise. Please avoid the sugary drinks that are branded to make them look like sports or performance drinks; they are nothing but sugar solutions.

Ultimately during a walk you should aim to drink at least 100ml every 10-15 minutes, especially if you are sweating. You should drink even if you do not feel particularly thirsty as there is no risk to consuming too much water, but too little can have adverse side effects and your performance will suffer, particularly if you are walking against the clock or in an event.

Eating salty-foods can also help tackle dehydration. Salt helps our body to absorb and retain water which will help you replace water lost through sweat. This is mostly important for ultra-long duration walks where you will need to schedule your meals in-between your periods of exercise.

As a side note, our body also needs salt for our nervous system as it is vital to creating the chemical conditions to produce the electrical signals that move our muscles. As a result if we lose too much salt through our sweat we can suffer from cramp. You can alleviate cramp caused by salt loss by drinking salt water or especially salty foods.

You should also learn to recognize the signs of dehydration. Obviously, when we are dehydrated we tend to become thirsty. However, most of us are poor at recognizing our own feelings of thirst. Often thirst is conflated with hunger or even just ignored altogether. Owing to this people often don't pay attention and can easily become dehydrated due to a lack of mindfulness.

Other symptoms of dehydration include dizziness, light-headedness, headaches, tiredness and dryness in the lips, mouth and eyes. In severe cases dehydration can cause severe lethargy, confusion, a weak or unstable pulse and a dizziness that doesn't pass when you stand upright.

These symptoms are caused by the brain and the blood being influenced by the lack of water. Our brains are composed of approximately 80% water and will start to condense and shrink when we are dehydrated, causing the symptoms of headaches, nausea, dizziness, tiredness and light-headedness.

Our blood will also lose volume, due to a lower water content, which places more pressure on the heart to compensate. This causes the changes in pulse and can contribute to tiredness as your body struggle to receive the oxygen and nutrients it needs through blood circulation.

In response the blood vessels dilate to try and allow more blood flow into vital areas, which causes swelling and inflammation. This causes an almost twofold attack on the brain – it shrinks due to the lack of water but is also inflamed and swollen due to blood vessel activity.

Walking & Nutrition

For both longer and shorter walks you should consider taking some food with you. For shorter walks a small energy rich sugary snack is recommended. Sugar has been made out to the enemy by the media, but as with most things in our diet, it is beneficial in moderation. Sugar is easily digestible and is one of the best ways for an instant energy kick, which is important for maintaining performance during intense exercise.

Of course the best foods to snack on contain natural sugars, such as dried fruits. Baked goods, candies and other human made sugary treats contain sugars in unhealthy proportions and are nutritionally devoid in other regards (such as their lack of fiber). We often see tennis players eating bananas between games at the side of the court; this is done as stated above to easily digest natural sugar for energy.

Fats slow down the digestion of sugar and can delay the release of energy. Therefore if you want a quick energy boost, avoid fatty foods. One un-expected source of fat can be the margarine and butter people use in sandwiches, which few people often consider.

For longer, slower walks fats can be beneficial due to their higher energy content and slower energy release, making them a better source of sustained energy. Good sources of fats can include healthy oils such as olive oil, although for walking, it is often most practical to stick with nuts and seeds, which are easy to carry and do not require a large amount of space.

However fats are also somewhat harder to digest than carbohydrates, so they should only be eaten in small amounts, especially for more intense periods of exercise.

Instead carbohydrate rich foods should be your primary source of energy. Carbohydrates (a category which includes sugars) are our body's primary source of energy and are easier to digest than proteins, fats and fiber. This makes them a better choice during exercise when our body has diverted energy away from digestive process and towards the muscles, respiratory and cardiovascular systems.

Chapter 3 –   Gear & Clothing

Pedometer

A pedometer is a device that tracks how many steps you have walked. It is typically worn on the ankle or the wrist, although some devices are attached to the hip. A pedometer doesn't have to be expensive, with many functional models retailing at less than $20, although sophisticated models can range all the way up to hundreds of dollars. Smart phones often have free apps worth looking at and usually you can find a really good pedometer app available to download for free. So try a few out until you find the one you really like.

It may be worth your while investing in a model that also tracks calorie expenditure and heart rate, although expect a degree of inaccuracy on the calorie count due the wide range of variables not accounted for (such as weight, gender, age, height, etc.).

Pedometers work by tracking the electronic pulses created by your movement when you walk. It's important to accurately input the length your typical step in, because this will influence the step count as well as other factors such as calorie count. It is important to refer to your device instructions here because some devices can use different terminology (such as stride instead of step) which can mislead you. When you have accurately established your step distance your pedometer will be able to estimate your total distance walked by multiplying your total steps by your step distance.

If you are walking for fitness, keep a log of the amount of steps and total distance you walk in each session in an excel spreadsheet or even in a notepad. This allows you to *know* just how far you have walked, so you can increment and adjust your walking patterns in a systematic way.

For many fitness walkers, an increase of 500 steps per week until they have reached a target step goal is a manageable increase to their overall amount of walking. Establishing a goal in terms of steps instead of total distance can be useful as it helps personalize the amount of effort to the effort required by your height.

A popular step goal is 10,000 steps per day, which equates to approximately 5 miles. Of course this is a generic goal and should be adjusted especially for the old or infirm.

You can also use a pedometer to track the total amount of steps you have walked during an entire day by wearing the device from the moment you wake up to the moment you fall asleep. This is helpful for several reasons. It gives you a baseline for the amount of exercise which you do every day without realizing, which may be more or less than you expect.

It also helps you incorporate small changes into your lifestyle to increase this count. Walking to work instead of driving, taking the stairs instead of the elevator, parking further away from your workplace and walking the remaining distance and numerous other small adjustments can increase your walking distance by a surprising amount.

Walking & Clothing

It's important to wear shoes that are comfortable and do not cause blisters when worn for longer durations. Shoes should also support your ankle and the sole of your foot, preventing minor injuries and strains. With that being said there is little need to buy and wear a pair of 'walking shoes' - any well-fitting, decent quality shoe should do.

You should also wear loose and comfortable clothes that allow you to move more freely and in a relaxed fashion. Tight clothes will cause sores when worn over long periods of time and may contribute to sweating and heat tiredness.
For especially long walks, consider taking sunglass with you as well as a sunhat and perhaps a spare shirt if you suspect that you may sweat extensively.

Walking Backpacks

For longer walks, you may want to bring a backpack with you. This ensures you have enough space for your drinks and snacks, but also important accessories such as sun cream, sunglass, medications, and your wallet and so on.

Choosing the right backpack is important. Too large and the backpack becomes too bothersome, too small and there isn't enough space. For the purpose of our fitness walking, you should prefer slightly smaller bags as you only need significant space for water, with all the other items included being rather small.

The distribution of weight is also a factor, with single-strap over the shoulder bags leading to back strain. Favor backpacks with two over the shoulder straps, but also connectors that bring around the chest and waist. This provides the optimal way to support the load and prevent any strain and aches. Backpacks with padded shoulder straps will help prevent the strap from digging into the shoulder and causing discomfort. It also helps distribute and balance the weight more evenly.

Also consider your weight. You should be able to adjust the straps on your backpack so that the straps and shoulder pads are in a comfortable position. Even if your backpack is of a good size and has all the right features, it is less useful if those features don't fit you.

Although the frequent call to prevent injury throughout this guide might seem rather excessive, it is important to realize just how easy it is for your body to become worn down over several weeks if precautions are not taken. You are unlikely to feel aches and strains during a single walk or shorts walks, but after hundreds of miles over numerous days and weeks, little strains and unnecessary burdens take their toll.

Ideally your backpack will also have a few external pockets that are easy to reach where you can store important accessible items such as water and snacks. If you have to stop, unzip and rummage through your backpack every time you want a drink or a bite to eat, it is easy to become a little frustrated with the effort. This can prevent some people from drinking enough water, leading to dehydration and the previously mentioned symptoms.

Some walkers even choose backpacks that have designated sections for large plastic filled bags of water and detachable straws that allow them to drink directly out of the bag. This might be a little over-the-top, but it is a fun possibility.

When choosing a backpack favor lightweight but sturdy materials over heavier and weaker materials. Leather bags and backpacks might be more fashionable, but all that extra weight will not be worth the style points.

A small portion of walkers chose to wear weighted backpacks to try and increase their calorie expenditure, a habit which is called rucking. Rucking is not recommended, however if you must include weights in your walking practice, it is a better choice than using ankle or wrist weights as it produces less strain on the smaller joints and tendons. Naturally if you have back problems, joint problems or muscle ache it is highly important to avoid using weights altogether, rucking or not.

It's important to invest in quality in regards to your backpack. A cheap backpack will last for a year; a good backpack will last for a lifetime.

Using a Treadmill

If you are self-conscious about fitness walking in public or lack a nearby area to freely walk in, consider investing in a treadmill. Walking on a treadmill provides all the same benefits as walking outdoors. In fact, walking on a treadmill is often better as you gain more precise control over several factors such as your incline and pace. Treadmills also provide fantastic tools to track your distance, heart rate and calorie expenditure. Furthermore they also tend to be a little easier on the joints and bones, at least compared to walking over concrete and asphalt in urban environments.

If you are interested in owning a treadmill, there are a few facts you need to consider. The first is price. It can be tempting to try and get the cheapest treadmill possible, but as the old adage goes, you get what you pay for. This is especially true for manual treadmills, which can be harder to use, less efficient and more prone to breaking.

Favor purchasing an electrical treadmill, preferably a DC treadmill. Electric treadmills can be AC or DC, but the former uses more electricity and produces more noise. Watch out for the quality of the belt that you run upon – thicker belters will endure for longer and tend to retain their shape whilst others deform. Similarly, higher quality belts also tend to be better at absorbing the impact of your walking, reducing strain on joints, tendons and bones. Of course, expect to pay more for these increases in belt thickness and quality.

Also be savvy and consider the size. Treadmills can be quite large, so it's important to accurately measure out the space you have available before committing to a purchase. Far too many people buy exercise equipment with the best intentions only to realize post-purchase that they do not have enough room or enjoy a more open feel to their household and therefore relegate the treadmill to the garage.

Larger sized treadmills can also be easier to use as they accommodate a wider gait as well as wider persons – you need to make sure you can comfortably fit inside the treadmill and walk on it freely.

Next, think about what other features you value. Fancy extras like a heart rate monitor, track setting and presets, calorie expenditure and more can be nice, but can also just add to the price without genuinely benefiting the quality of your workout. Generally speaking, practical design benefits are the most important factors – a place to rest a drink for example, hold a sweat towel, rest a TV or place your MP3 are probably all more important than electronic features.

Overall if you are committed to making walking a hobby, be prepared to part with a sizeable chunk of your cash to get a high quality treadmill. Expect to pay more than a few hundred dollars; although the higher prices might be intimidating, the cheaper specimens are a lesson in false economy. Of course, research the brand and style of the treadmill you intend to buy in advance as price might be misleading – your retailer might just be selling overpriced units.

That being said walking is a brilliant pastime that can be performed without the need for fancy expensive equipment. We would only recommend purchasing the above as an absolute last resort or if injury restricts you from walking in the great outdoors.

Chapter 4 - Injury & Prevention

Healthy Knees

Although walking is less strenuous on the joints than other forms of exercise, it can still contribute to joint problems, especially when walking for longer distances. Furthermore as walking uses certain joints excessively, it can focus the strain of exercise in just a few particular areas, such as the knees.

To avoid joint problems it is important to incrementally increase your level of exercise. If you are attempting to achieve 10,000 steps per day, try to gradually increase your steps in small amounts until you reach that goal.

You should also consider your walking technique. We rarely think about walking in terms of technique, but there are some methods of walking that are more efficient and less strenuous than others.

For example one bad habit when walking is called *overpronation*. When we walk the sole of our foot rolls against the ground slightly to absorb the impact of our foot against the floor and balance our weight. Overpronation is the habit of rolling the sole of your foot too much when you walk, rather than pushing off the ground for the next step, which causes your weight to be resting on just one side of your foot. Overpronation bends the foot, the calf and the knee and can lead to pain and tiredness in these areas.

One tell-tale sign of overpronation is the wear of your shoes; if your shoes are worn down on the inner side, you may overpronate. You can correct this habit by paying more attention to your stride as you walk, but also consider buying corrective shoes to help adjust your technique. Shoes with straight or semi-curved lasts can help combat this habit, whilst specific arch supports or motion-control shoes are also useful.

Stretching can also help relax the muscles, which can reduce the tendency to overpronate during walking.

Underpronation, also known as supination, is the opposite; the foot doesn't roll enough to absorb the impact, concentrating the impact of collision against the outer areas of the foot, which also stresses the joints in the legs and the feet. If you underpronate, your shoes should also be unevenly worn, but on the outer edge.

For underpronators, shoes with curved lasts will help correct your bad habit. You should also favor lighter and more flexible material for your shoes as these allow for more motion, making it easier to pronate correctly.

If you still find that you have aches and pains in your legs, ankles and feet following a walking session, consider the ground you walk upon. Harder, uneven or slippery surface are more difficult to walk over and may cause excess strain. Therefore, if possible, try to avoid surfaces like concrete or asphalt and instead try and walk over grassy or earthy areas, which absorb the impact of your feet better. The local park is a great place to walk. Likewise avoid walking over sand or snow which requires more effort.

Shoes should be replaced on a semi-frequent basis. The protective aspects of shoes will be degraded through prolonged walking, especially the inner support, increasing the risk of injury and other problems. A good ballpark is that shoes should be replaced between every 300 – 500 miles. If you have a hard time calculating how this number equates to steps or distance, it equates to around 6 months of time for someone walking approximately 10,000 steps per day.

It can be useful to purchase multiple pairs of walking shoes to rotate between in case one pair gets damaged and can no longer be used (or for any reason is no longer usable).

Stretching & Warm Up

Even though walking is perceived as a milder form of exercise than running or most sports, it can still be useful to stretch and warm up before you have a walking session. Nonetheless, successful stretching and warming up reduces injury and muscle fatigue and can increase performance during a particular session. Warming up increases the blood flow to your muscles - this prepares them for a greater level of activity.

Common warm-up stretches for walking include:

Calf Stretches: Stand upright, grasping a chair or a piece of furniture to keep you steady. Take a step back with your left leg, keeping the heel of your foot on the floor. Bend your right knee, leaning your body towards the furniture. As you place your weight forward you should feel the stretch in your left leg. Hold this pose for several moments, repeating the movement with the legs in the opposite positions.

Hamstring & Ankle: Sit on the edge of a chair. Move your right leg forward on the floor, ensuring the heel still touches the floor. Flex your right foot, ensuring that your keep your toes pointing directly as the sky. Learn your torso and upper body forward, until a stretch is felt in the thigh. Hold this posture for a moment before repeating with the legs in the alternate position.

Groin Stretch: Stand upright with your legs slightly further than shoulder length apart grasping a chair or piece of furniture in front of you. Pivot your feet so that your left foot is pointing forward whilst you right foot is pointing at a 45 degree angle. Lunge with the right foot, ensuring that the knee doesn't surpass the feet. Repeat the feet in the other positions.

Leg Swings: Stand upright, grasping a chair or piece of furniture to the side of your body. Grasp it with your nearest hand. Move your left leg forward, then to the side of your body, then behind, taping the floor with your toes at each point. Repeat with the alternate leg.

Cooling Down

It's just as important to cool down as it is to warm up! Cooling down allows your heartbeat and muscles to acclimatize to a lower level of activity, which can take several minutes after an intense bout of exercise. If your body changes for intense exercise to sedentary levels of activity too quickly, it can actually stress the body – which is why athletes will often perform a gentle jog after finishing their exercise.

To cool down, simply gradually slow your walking over the period of several moments, allowing your heartbeat to decline steadily.

Using Weights

Many people try and use hand or ankle weights to add resistance to their walking routine. This is not recommended. Generally speaking it is incredibly difficult to add enough weight to build up muscle. However, this is not the reason why it is discouraged by the walking community – the strain weights place upon the ankle as well as the pressure on tendons, ligaments and blood pressure may result in injury.

Furthermore, people who wear weights tend to walker slower, removing any calorie burn effect that the extra weight might produce. Instead of adding weights, if you want to make your walk more intense, try walking with a faster pace. Alternatively, introduce weights into your lifestyle in a formal and controlled way in the gym. Resistance training with carefully considered repetitions will build up muscle strength and mass with more consistency and ease than slapping a few weights around your ankles and wrists.

Walking & Posture

When walking it is important to maintain proper posture. Your head should be upright and centered rather than leaning forwards, backwards or towards either of your shoulders. Likewise your chin should stay parallel to the ground, with a raised or sagged chin putting excess strain on the neck.

If you suspect that you do not keep your head upright or your chin parallel to the ground, try balancing a flat object on your head such as a book or folder. If the object stays balanced without any support your head is in the correct position – if not, your posture could use improvement. Of course the objective isn't to go outside balancing objects on your head, it is simply to get a sense of how a good posture should feel.

Your shoulders should also be relaxed. As a result of stress or merely chronic bad habits many people raise and tense their shoulders whilst walking. This can contribute to pain and stiffness in the shoulders, but also prevent a natural walking rhythm, making walking harder.

Conversely the chest should be lifted and expanded. You don't have to walk around like a puffin, but your chest should be raised as this helps straighten the back. If you have a hard time envisioning what a raised chest should feel like, imagine that you are being pulled upwards by a rope from the center of your ribcage – this should be your walking posture, all of the time!

However, correct posture concerns more than just the upper body - whilst walking you should also gently tense your abdominal muscles. This helps keep the lower spine straight. Of course you won't be able to breathe or walk easily if you strongly contract your abdominal muscles, so don't over-do it.

Additionally, your buttocks should also be directly below your hips. If you are leaning forward and not properly supporting your back, your buttocks will stick out from the rest of your body.

Also, whilst walking you need to ensure you arms have a natural and fluid swing in response to your movement. If your elbows are tensed or if you are holding your arms in towards your torso you will inhibit this motion, so ensure you attempt to relax and allow your body to move how it wants to.

Finally, also consider your walking stride. The length of your stride should vary according to your weight, the flexibility of your hips and the stiffness of the muscles in your leg. It is a good idea to experiment with different walking strides and get a sense of what feels most natural and efficient.

Common Walking Injuries and Solutions

We have talked a lot about preventing injuries, but no matter how careful you are, at some point you are likely to experience some type of walking injury. Therefore it can be useful to understand, distinguish and appreciate the different common injuries that occur so you can learn to recover from them sooner.

Plantar Fasciitis

The plantar fasciitis is the tissue at the base of your foot which connects your heel and ball of your feet. The main use of this tissue is to absorb and disperse the impact and shock of walking and running. If your technique is poor or you over-exert yourself your plantar fasciitis can become torn and stretched, resulting in tenderness and soreness at the base of the foot. Tears in the plantar fasciitis are particularly common from running on the pavement and hard concrete which do not absorb or disperse any of the shock of impact themselves.

To help cope and prevent plantar fasciitis injuries pay attention to any stiffness or tenderness at the base of the foot. When feeling tender, stretch that area by sitting down, extending the leg and pulling the toes and ball of the foot until you feel a stretch in the arch of the foot. Repeat this several times for both feet until the tissue has loosened.

Bunions

Bunions are caused when the joints in the toes become skewed and do not connect to each other cleanly. This causes swelling and inflammation in the area, eventually forming a bunion. Some people are more likely to form bunions than others, especially people who have arthritis, or especially flat feet.

If you are susceptible to bunions, invest in a wide pair of shoes. Wider pairs of shoes can allow you to fit pads and protective gear inside the shoes reducing pressure on the bunion and also lowering friction. Bunions are complicated to treat and they may require therapy or surgery to realign the joints into the correct position.

Achilles Tendonitis

Essentially pain in your calf and your heel, Achilles tendinitis is simply caused by over-exertion, especially if there is not a suitable period of warming up and stretching before exercise. It can also be caused if the foot flexes too much whilst moving due to sharp inclines or uneven ground.

Reducing the length of your walking distance, improving your warm-up periods and running on even, flat ground are all good choices for combating Achilles tendonitis.

If the pain is severe, consider stopping your exercise regime until the condition has improved and using ice packs to help battle inflammation. When the condition has improved, return to your previous intensity and distance of walking or exercise gradually, allowing your muscle to re-adjust.

Lower Back Pain

Lower back pain is caused by poor walking technique. It is unlikely to result purely from walking, but walking may exacerbate the back pain caused by chronic poor posture, being overweight or previous back injury.

Keeping your spine upright and tightening your abs whilst you walk are the best solutions to lower back pain. You can try to straighten your back by raising your arms vertically above your head and pushing upwards.

Shin Splints

Whilst you are standing upright your shins bear a great weight load compared to other positions and this is especially true for running and walking. Shin splints are caused by the muscles in the calf and surrounding areas being too weak to suddenly deal with a greater level of activity caused by walking and running.

Lowering your level of activity can help shin splints improve whilst anti-inflammatory and pain relief medication can deal with other symptoms. Also consider specific exercises to strengthen and tone your calves, such as calf raises or squats.

Using runners tape can also help with shin splints. Any good sports store or online store should stock runners tape. Simply apply the tape to your shins or how instructed on the packaging.

Bursitis

Bursitis is soreness and inflammation around the hips. For most of the joints in our body, fluid-filled sacs help cushion and absorb impact in the joint sockets, preventing wear and tear of the bones. Injury is often caused by these sacs bursting or being destroyed but in the case of bursitis, the fluid-filled sacs become inflamed and swell. Bursitis is caused by excessive stress, usually caused by a rapid increase in activity and effort.

To help deal with bursitis you should vary your exercise regime with forms of exercise where your weight isn't being rested on the legs, such as swimming or cycling. You can also consider lowering your overall level of activity.

Bursitis can also be prevented by gradually increasing your level of activity rather than sudden and large increases. Likewise when overcoming bursitis gradually return to your former level of activity otherwise you might experience a relapse in symptoms.

Ingrown Toenails

Ingrown toenails occur when the toenails themselves bend and grow into the surrounding flesh. Ingrown toenails can be incredibly painful and even cause the toenail to be ripped away from the toe. Not only is this excruciating, but toenails don't always grow back, leading to permanent damage to your foot!

Ingrown toenails are predominantly caused by shoes that are too small, especially width-wise. As a result, buying roomier shoes can help solve the condition. Likewise keeping your toenails neatly trimmed and preventing them from growing too long also helps.

Neuroma

Neuroma is recognized by the pain it caused in the ball of the foot and the toes. Neuroma is actually caused by the nerves in the foot growing and thickening altering the sensations in the foot – it can also produce numbness or an unpleasant tingling.

Neuroma is by far more common in women than in men, although the exact reason is not known. However it has been hypothesized that this gender-difference may be caused due to the structure of the female foot and the tendency for women to wear punishing and poorly fitting shoes, such as high heels.

Neuroma can be improved by wearing shoes that fit better and balance the weight evenly across the foot. However it's important to immediately consult a doctor if you suspect you are suffering from Neuroma as the condition can progress rapidly.

Chapter 5 – Long Distance Walking & Race Walking

Walking a Marathon

If you are ambitious, walking a marathon is a great way to push your fitness and walking habits further. You will need to train and schedule your walks to gradually improve your fitness and timing until you are able to complete a marathon within the designated time.

Most training plans for marathon walking start by aiming to walk between 15-20 miles in a single week. This prepares your body to walk long distances semi-frequently and ensures that you are less likely to develop injury or become fatigued as your training program intensifies.

It takes time for the body to adapt to regular exercise, even for walking. The longer and more forgiving your marathon training is the better. If you are someone who is sedentary, try aiming to build up your walking practice over the course of several months *before* you begin training for a marathon. It just takes that long for your muscles to grow and joints and tendons to adapt.

The better walking programs try to walk between 4-6 days a week. You want to walk regularly and ensure you walk a large amount of miles, but still have a few days of the week where your body gets to relax and recuperate.

You can also stagger your walking and experiment with different paces. For your regular walking it is best to maintain a consistent pace throughout the entire walk – fast enough to challenge yourself, easy enough to stay at for long periods of time.

However you can also add interval walking into your practice, where you alternate between a comfortable natural pace and a fast, brisk walk. This helps build up your recovery from intense periods of exercise and it also helps you acclimatize, psychologically, to harder levels of activity. Try five minutes of walking at a natural pace followed by five minutes of walking at a brisk pace.

You can walk on your recovery days, but your focus should not be on fitness or calorie burn but instead comfortable and gentle walking. You should also use the more relaxed pace of the walk to focus more on the form and technique of your walking whilst you walk.

Additionally, you can also add a long-distance day to your walk. The pace of this walk should be above a comfortable pace, but nor should it be strenuous. Long distance is useful to build up stamina. Gradually over the course of several months you should increase the speed of your long distance walk until you have achieved the walking pace you want to replicate during your marathon.

Also consider adding a cross training session to your walking schedule. A cross training session can be incredibly similar in intensity and calorie burn to your walking session, but it uses different muscles and places less pressure on the joints, bones and tendons. Therefore it is good to slip in between your more intense walking periods as a way to keep your level of activity high but give your body some degree of rest.

To summarize for a 4-6 day schedule of marathon walking try to do the following:
1 day of regular walking
1 day of interval day
1 day of fast walking
1 day of long distance
1 cross training session
1 recovery walk

And, of course, it's also important to have at least one day where you give your body a complete rest. Finally as the date of the actual marathon arrives, you need to taper off and decrease your level of activity. This sounds counter-intuitive, but it is in fact important for optimal performance. When undergoing a marathon you want your muscles and body to be in peak condition. If you have kept up your exercise program religiously, your muscles will be tired and your energy stores depleted when it comes to the actual marathon. Therefore you need to give yourself a grace period of 1-2 weeks before the marathon where you exercise less intensely and limit yourself to slower and shorter walks.

Long-Distance Walking

In the previous sections of this guide, the emphasis has mostly been directed towards short and moderate walking distances. However many runners enjoy the challenge of huge walking distances – distances so long that they must be walked over days and weeks rather than minutes and hours. This section provides advice and guidance on how to complete these ultra-long walks.

For walking over long distances, consider wearing two or more pairs of socks to help reduce friction. However, your feet must still have room to move. In fact your feet actually expand as you walk, due to blood pressure dilation and continued pressure of the weight of your body, so extra room is essential.

It can also be a good idea to keep spare pairs of socks with you in case you need to change along the walk – keeping your feet dry helps prevent a wide array of problems. Although wearing lighter trainers will tire your legs less, boots can be a better choice for longer walks, especially over unstable ground, to reduce the chances of hurting your ankle.

Psychology and motivation starts to become important for long distance walkers. Segment your long distance walk into chunks that feel more achievable – 1 mile, 5 miles, 10 miles and so on. This can be used for smaller distances too – 10 strides, 100 strides, the next lamppost and so on.

If you start to flag and feel like you can't continue just focus on the immediate moment – take it literally one step at a time. Reward yourself for the milestones you do complete, allowing yourself to feel a sense of accomplishment for every segment of your walk that you do complete. Try not to think of the challenge before you as realizing that you still have 20 miles or 50 miles before you can be overwhelming. Most of us chronically underestimate our own abilities and will feel like we simply cannot achieve our goal once we start to struggle. Yet ruminating, brooding and worrying won't improve your internal battle – keep your mind clear and on task.

It can also help to have company, as a little humor to lift your spirits can go a long way. Even if your friends and colleagues lack a flair for comedy, conversation can help keep the mind distracted from the small aches and pains that are bound to arise over such long distances.

Keeping your feet in good condition is vital during a challenging long-distance walk. You must learn how to take preventative measures to prevent small blisters and sores from becoming worse. If you think you are starting to develop a blister for example, you should ensure that you cover the area with a plaster or *moleskin,* a type of fabric popular among walkers to help reduce friction.

You also need to keep your feet dry at all times. An especially problem among long-distances walkers is trench foot, which is where the feet become white, waxy and crinkled. Essentially trench foot is the same process that occurs when you spend too long in the bathtub and your hands become wrinkly, just in this instance to your feet. This is caused by the feet constantly being wet and it can lead to a lot of damage of the skin and be very uncomfortable.

Apart from keeping your shoes and socks dry, you can also help combat trench foot through Vaseline and water-repellent grease to help keep a protective layer between your shoes and socks, and your skin.

Another good piece of advice is to neatly trim and cut your toenails. Long toenails will continually rub against your shoes and socks and become painful. Your toenail may even break away from the toe altogether, which is very painful and a persistent issue for long distance walkers.

During long walks you need to eat an extraordinary amount of food. Walking is often considered a less-calorie intensive form of exercise compared to most activities, but the opposite is true for long distance walks. For an average person an hour of walking burns approximately 300 calories. Therefore if you walk for an entire day you can easily burn 2000-2500 calories just from walking, without counting any extra calories you need for warmth, carrying weight and basic processes to keep you alive.

Therefore during long walks you need to focus on bringing calorie rich food with you such as dried fruit, isotonic drinks and even the occasional treat, such as chocolate. Furthermore you also need to force yourself to eat, even if you don't feel like it. During exercise our body diverts energy and attention away from the digestive systems and towards the muscles, with often causes the signals for hunger not to be produced, even if you need the energy. Ultimately if you fail to eat enough, it will catch up with you after a few hours or few days. Favor frequent but smaller meals, which are easier to digest and supply you with a more consistent stream of energy.

In extreme cases people may struggle to stomach food without vomiting, nausea or severe discomfort. If you find this happening to you, try to consume energy rich drinks. Some walkers also find success with weird but easily palatable high-energy foods, such as custard.

You should also be aware of the possibility of hypothermia, especially due to the harsh conditions you may be placing yourself in. If your body is primarily using energy for walking, it may have difficulty producing enough heat to keep you warm. Likewise if you walk during the evening the temperature can drop rapidly and become incredibly cool, even during the summer months.

Therefore you need clothing that is suitable. Your clothes should retain heat both from the wind and but also when they are wet, which tends to limit your choices to wool or thermals. Even if you only feel a slightly chill it is a good idea to wrap another layer on.

For long distance walking it is best to walk at a comfortable pace. If the walking pace you are maintaining is uncomfortable that means you are exerting yourself, which also means you will struggle to maintain that pace over a long period of time.

Race Walking

Race walking is a sporting competition where competitors walk anywhere between 3km to 100km. It is an Olympic sport and has existed almost as long the modern Olympics itself, being first added to the competition in 1908.

Race walking has some interesting rules. Although the sport is called *race* walking, the winner isn't always necessarily the fastest contestant. Rather performance is judged by race walking judges who evaluate factors such as speed but also technique. During the race contestants are strictly limited to walking and walking only, with jogging or running in any form leading to penalties. Walking is defined as movement where the back toe cannot leave the ground until the heel of the forward foot has touched the ground.

Another important rule is the supporting leg – the leg with the foot currently touching the floor - must remain touching the floor and straighten whilst the body moves over it, giving race walking a distinctive technique.

To help maintain this technique, race walkers typically keep their arms lower to the ground than conventional walkers, around their hips rather than their torso. This lower positioning of the arms ensures that there is no upward swing or motion causing the feet to leave the ground simultaneously, breaking the rules of race walking technique.

Instead of airborne strides, race walkers use fast and frequent smaller steps as well as pelvic movement that ensure they propel forward at speed. This is achieved by pushing sharply upwards from the ball of the foot.

Race walking can achieve rather impressive speeds for walking. Top race walkers can reach around 4 minutes per kilometer and maintain this distance over a few dozen miles. However this speed requires an extreme degree of fitness and technique – don't expect to reach this level quickly.

Race walking is a great way to challenge your fitness through walking, especially if you lack the time and resources to commit to long-distance walking challenges. It's important to emphasize here that race walking is a real and demanding sport; don't expect it to be easy, even if you are an advanced walker or runner. Many athletes in other sports comment on how hard race walking can be both from a physical and a mental perspective. Race walking requires a constant focus on technique, which requires a deep and persistent attention span.

It also requires openness and a blank slate to walking technique. If you try to start race walking with preconceived notions of how fast you can walk or how far you can go, you will often find yourself much more limited and much slower to progress than you may anticipate. When you start race walking your focus should purely be upon correct technique, which often translates to walking slowly and for limited distances. However once you have proficient techniques you can rapidly upscale increase the duration and length of your walks.

Conclusion

Walking is fun, free and improves fitness. It carries significantly lower risk of injury than other forms of exercise and it is easier to develop into a habit and sustain than most other forms of activity. I hope this guide has helped you develop walking into a life changing and positive part of your lifestyle.

Remember that walking is a fun and easy way to gain some level of basic fitness. It also has the benefit of being something that we all do to varying degrees every day throughout our waking hours.

Just take a walk to the local shops instead of taking the car or bus. Just doing this once a week will have you fitter than you would have otherwise been if you hadn't.

So get your shoes on and go for a walk. You won't regret it!

Most of all………

………enjoy it!!!

Faye Froome

Made in the USA
Middletown, DE
21 December 2021

56777952R00031